Endometriosis

Women's Reproductive Health

Complete Resource for Understanding and Managing Endometriosis with Pain Relief, Fertility Support, and Surgical Treatment Options

Graham Julian Oliver

Disclaimer

The information provided in this book, *Epilepsy – A Neurological Disorder Characterized by Recurrent Seizures: In-Depth Guide to Managing Epilepsy with Seizure Control, Medication, and Long-Term Treatment Strategies for Neurological Health*, is intended for informational purposes only. It is not a substitute for professional medical advice, diagnosis, or treatment. Always seek the advice of your physician or other qualified health provider with any questions you may have regarding a medical condition or treatment.

The author and publisher do not endorse any individual, product, website, organization, or other names mentioned in this book. All references included are solely for informational purposes and do not imply any endorsement or recommendation. Reliance on any information provided in this book is solely at your own risk.

While the author has made every effort to provide accurate and up-to-date information, there may be errors or omissions. The author and publisher disclaim any liability for any direct or indirect loss or damage resulting from the use or reliance on the information contained herein.

Disclaimer

The information provided in this book, *Endometriosis – Women's Reproductive Health: Complete Resource for Understanding and Managing Endometriosis with Pain Relief, Fertility Support, and Surgical Treatment Options*, is intended for informational purposes only and should not be considered a substitute for professional medical advice, diagnosis, or treatment. Always seek the advice of your physician or other qualified health provider with any questions you may have regarding a medical condition.

The author does not make any representations or warranties about the completeness, reliability, or accuracy of the information contained in this book. Any reliance you place on such information is strictly at your own risk. The author is not liable for any losses or damages in connection with the use of this book.

Furthermore, the author does not endorse or have any affiliation with any individual, product, website, organization, or other names mentioned or referenced in this book. Any mention of such entities is solely for informational purposes. The inclusion of these references does not imply endorsement or recommendation by the author.

By reading this book, you acknowledge that you have read and understood this disclaimer and agree to its terms.

About This Book

The book titled **Endometriosis — Women's Reproductive Health** serves as a vital resource for women navigating the complex journey of understanding and managing endometriosis. This comprehensive guide provides a thorough overview of endometriosis, shedding light on its definition, development, symptoms, and various stages. It emphasizes the critical importance of awareness and education, highlighting how knowledge can empower women to recognize and respond to their symptoms effectively. This foundational understanding is essential, as early detection plays a crucial role in managing the condition and mitigating its impact on daily life.

The impact of endometriosis extends far beyond physical symptoms; it significantly affects women's emotional and psychological well-being. This book addresses the often-overlooked emotional challenges associated with the condition, advocating for the necessity of support networks and resources. By fostering an environment of understanding and compassion, women can find strength in community, making it easier to navigate the unique challenges that endometriosis presents. This emphasis on emotional health is vital, as it empowers women to seek help and share their experiences, ultimately promoting a more informed and supportive society around this condition.

Pain management strategies are a central focus of this resource, offering an array of options that range from over-the-counter medications to non-pharmacological techniques. The book provides valuable insights into the role of lifestyle changes, mindfulness, and nutritional considerations in alleviating pain. By presenting a multifaceted approach to pain relief, it encourages women to create individualized pain management plans that cater to their unique needs and circumstances. Furthermore, the connection between endometriosis and fertility is explored in depth, providing essential information about how the condition can affect reproductive health. This includes a discussion of fertility tests, treatment options, and emotional considerations, ensuring that women feel supported and informed as they navigate their fertility journeys.

Surgical treatment options are also discussed comprehensively, equipping readers with knowledge about the various types of surgeries available, their indications, and what to expect throughout the surgical process. Understanding potential risks and the importance of choosing a skilled surgeon can help women make informed decisions about their care. Post-surgery recovery tips and the significance of follow-up care are highlighted, ensuring that readers are prepared for their journey after surgical intervention.

Moreover, the role of nutrition and lifestyle modifications is underscored throughout the book. The relationship between diet and endometriosis symptoms is explored, offering practical advice on anti-inflammatory foods and nutritional supplements that can contribute to better health. This holistic approach emphasizes the importance of incorporating healthy habits into daily life, addressing factors such as hydration, exercise, and stress management. By equipping women with the tools to make informed lifestyle choices, the book empowers them to take an active role in their health management.

Emotional and psychological support is given due consideration, as the book delves into counseling options, stress reduction techniques, and the importance of building a robust support system. The significance of self-care, journaling, and advocacy are also emphasized, encouraging women to seek empowerment through shared experiences and active participation in raising awareness about endometriosis. By fostering a sense of community and shared advocacy, the book helps women understand their rights in healthcare and the importance of engaging with advocacy organizations.

Living well with endometriosis is a central theme of the book, encouraging readers to develop personalized management plans that accommodate their unique situations. It addresses the importance of routine check-ups and long-term planning, emphasizing resilience and coping skills. By highlighting common concerns and providing detailed FAQs, the resource offers a well-rounded understanding of endometriosis, addressing questions about diagnosis, treatment options, lifestyle changes, and emotional support.

In essence, this book serves as a comprehensive and empowering resource for women facing the challenges of endometriosis. By providing in-depth knowledge and practical tools, it fosters a sense of agency and community, allowing women to navigate their journeys with confidence and clarity. This vital resource stands as a testament to the importance of understanding, managing, and advocating for women's reproductive health.

Table of Contents

Introduction
Definition and Overview of Endometriosis

Endometriosis is a chronic condition where tissue similar to the lining of the uterus, called endometrial tissue, grows outside the uterus. This tissue can be found on the ovaries, fallopian tubes, and other areas within the pelvis. During the menstrual cycle, this tissue thickens, breaks down, and bleeds, leading to inflammation, pain, and the formation of scar tissue. Symptoms can vary widely but commonly include pelvic pain, heavy menstrual bleeding, and discomfort during intercourse. Understanding these symptoms is crucial for early diagnosis and management.

To diagnose endometriosis, healthcare providers may conduct a pelvic exam, ultrasound, or laparoscopy—a surgical procedure that allows direct visualization of the pelvic organs. The exact cause of endometriosis remains unclear, but factors like genetics, immune system disorders, and hormonal influences may play a role. It's essential for individuals experiencing symptoms to seek medical advice, as timely diagnosis can help in managing the condition effectively and reducing its impact on quality of life.

Importance of Awareness and Education about the Condition

Raising awareness and educating both the public and healthcare professionals about endometriosis is vital for improving diagnosis rates and treatment options. Many individuals with endometriosis suffer in silence due to a lack of understanding of their symptoms or the belief that painful periods are normal. Education initiatives can empower those affected by the condition to seek help and advocate for their health. Additionally, educating healthcare providers can lead to more accurate and timely diagnoses, ensuring that patients receive appropriate care.

Engaging in awareness campaigns, community support groups, and social media platforms can foster a supportive environment for those affected by endometriosis. These resources provide valuable information on managing symptoms, coping strategies, and connecting with others who share similar experiences. Increasing awareness can also encourage research funding, ultimately leading to better treatments and possibly a cure for this challenging condition.

The Impact of Endometriosis on Women's Lives

Emotional and Psychological Effects of Endometriosis

Endometriosis not only impacts physical health but also significantly affects emotional and psychological well-being. Many women with endometriosis experience feelings of isolation, anxiety, and depression due to chronic pain and the unpredictability of their symptoms. These emotional challenges can exacerbate the physical aspects of the condition, leading to a cycle of pain and distress. Recognizing these emotional effects is crucial, as they can influence daily functioning, relationships, and overall quality of life.

To manage these emotional challenges, women are encouraged to seek mental health support, whether through therapy, support groups, or counseling. Developing coping strategies such as mindfulness, journaling, and engaging in creative outlets can also help alleviate stress. Furthermore, communicating openly with loved ones about feelings and experiences can foster understanding and support, helping to create a more nurturing environment.

Importance of Support and Resources for Women with Endometriosis

Having a strong support network is vital for women managing endometriosis. Support groups, whether online or in-person, provide a space to share experiences, challenges, and coping strategies with others facing similar issues. Connecting with fellow women who understand the daily struggles of endometriosis can reduce feelings of isolation and offer emotional comfort, making the journey more manageable.

Additionally, accessing reliable resources—such as educational materials, local healthcare providers, and holistic health practitioners—can empower women to take control of their health. Utilizing these resources can facilitate informed discussions with healthcare providers, enabling women to advocate for appropriate treatments and support tailored to their needs. Regularly seeking information and connecting with supportive communities can significantly enhance the overall management of endometriosis.

CHAPTER 1:

What is Endometriosis?

How Endometriosis Develops

Endometriosis occurs when tissue similar to the lining of the uterus grows outside it, commonly on the ovaries, fallopian tubes, and pelvic lining. This tissue responds to hormonal changes during the menstrual cycle, leading to inflammation, pain, and scar tissue formation. Factors like retrograde menstruation, where menstrual blood flows backward through the fallopian tubes, and immune system disorders are believed to contribute to the development of this condition.

To understand the development process, consider the role of hormones, particularly estrogen. During menstruation, the tissue outside the uterus thickens and sheds, similar to the uterine lining. However, unlike the lining, this tissue has no way to exit the body, causing inflammation and pain. Recognizing the hormonal aspect is key to grasping how endometriosis progresses and affects the body.

Common Symptoms to Watch For

Women with endometriosis often experience a range of symptoms, the most common being pelvic pain, which may occur during menstruation, intercourse, or bowel movements. Other symptoms can include heavy menstrual bleeding, fatigue, and gastrointestinal issues such as diarrhea or constipation. It's crucial to track these symptoms as they can help in understanding the severity and impact on daily life.

Keeping a symptom diary can be a practical tool for recognizing patterns. Note when symptoms occur, their intensity, and any potential triggers. This information can be invaluable during medical consultations, allowing healthcare providers to better assess the situation and develop effective management strategies.

Different Stages of Endometriosis

Endometriosis is classified into four stages: minimal, mild, moderate, and severe, based on the extent of the tissue growth and the presence of adhesions. Stage I (minimal) has small implants, while Stage IV (severe) presents with deep, large lesions and significant adhesions. Understanding these stages helps women identify their condition's severity and inform treatment decisions.

Women can discuss these stages with their healthcare provider during diagnosis. This conversation should focus on the specific characteristics of their endometriosis, as well as possible treatment options based on the stage. Knowing the stage can aid in creating personalized management plans.

Risk Factors Associated with the Condition

Certain risk factors may increase the likelihood of developing endometriosis, including family history, early menstruation, short menstrual cycles, and prolonged estrogen exposure. Additionally, lifestyle factors like high body weight and low physical activity may also play a role. Recognizing these risk factors can empower women to take proactive steps in managing their reproductive health.

To mitigate these risks, women should consider lifestyle changes, such as maintaining a healthy weight through a balanced diet and regular exercise. Regular check-ups with healthcare providers can also help monitor reproductive health, especially for those with a family history of endometriosis.

How Endometriosis Is Diagnosed

Diagnosing endometriosis typically involves a combination of pelvic exams, imaging tests like ultrasounds, and laparoscopy, a minimally invasive surgical procedure. During laparoscopy, a surgeon can view the pelvic organs and, if necessary, take biopsies for further examination. It's important for women to advocate for themselves if they suspect endometriosis, as it can sometimes be overlooked.

For those experiencing persistent symptoms, seeking a second opinion can be beneficial. Discussing symptoms openly with a healthcare provider and expressing concerns about endometriosis can lead to appropriate diagnostic measures, ensuring a comprehensive evaluation.

Importance of Early Detection

Early detection of endometriosis is crucial for effective management and improving quality of life. Women who recognize symptoms early are more likely to receive timely treatment, which can help alleviate pain and address fertility concerns. Additionally, early intervention can prevent the progression of the disease and the development of severe symptoms.

Women should prioritize regular gynecological check-ups and maintain open communication with their healthcare providers about any changes in their reproductive health. Staying informed and proactive can significantly enhance outcomes related to endometriosis management.

Impact on Daily Life

Endometriosis can profoundly affect daily life, influencing physical activities, work performance, and emotional well-being. Women may experience debilitating pain, fatigue, and mental health challenges, leading to missed work or social engagements. Understanding this impact is essential for developing effective coping strategies and seeking support.

To navigate these challenges, women are encouraged to build a support network, including friends, family, and healthcare professionals. Self-care practices, such as mindfulness, stress management, and regular exercise, can also help improve overall well-being and reduce the emotional toll of the condition.

Myths and Misconceptions

There are many myths surrounding endometriosis, including misconceptions that it only affects women who are infertile or that it always presents with severe pain. Such misconceptions can lead to stigma and misunderstandings, preventing women from seeking the help they need. Education and awareness are vital to dispelling these myths.

To combat misinformation, women should seek reliable sources of information, such as healthcare providers or reputable organizations dedicated to reproductive health. Engaging in discussions about endometriosis can help raise awareness and foster a more supportive environment for those affected.

Connection between Endometriosis and Other Health Issues

Endometriosis is often linked to other health issues, such as infertility, ovarian cysts, and autoimmune disorders. Understanding these connections can help women recognize the broader implications of their condition and encourage comprehensive healthcare. It's important for women to discuss these potential associations with their healthcare providers.

Maintaining a holistic view of health can aid in addressing related concerns. Women may benefit from integrative approaches that consider both endometriosis and any associated health issues, ensuring a more thorough management plan that addresses overall well-being.

Current Statistics and Prevalence

Endometriosis affects an estimated 1 in 10 women of reproductive age, highlighting its significance as a widespread condition. Awareness of these statistics can encourage women to seek help and validate their experiences, knowing they are not alone. Understanding the prevalence can also support advocacy efforts for better research and treatment options.

Women can use these statistics to raise awareness in their communities and advocate for greater resources and research funding. Sharing personal stories and statistics can help break the silence surrounding endometriosis and promote a more supportive environment for those affected.

Resources for Further Learning

Numerous resources are available for women seeking to learn more about endometriosis. Reputable organizations, books, and online forums can provide valuable information and support. These resources can empower women to understand their condition better and connect with others facing similar challenges.

Exploring local support groups or online communities can also foster a sense of belonging and provide opportunities for sharing experiences. Engaging with these resources can enhance knowledge and offer practical advice for managing endometriosis.

Importance of Patient Advocacy

Patient advocacy is crucial for women with endometriosis to ensure they receive the appropriate care and support. Being informed about their rights and options enables women to actively participate in their healthcare decisions. Advocacy can lead to better treatment outcomes and increased awareness about the condition.

Women can become advocates by educating themselves and others about endometriosis, sharing their experiences, and participating in awareness campaigns. Collaborating with healthcare professionals and organizations can help amplify their voices and push for necessary changes in endometriosis research and treatment.

CHAPTER 2:

Recognizing Symptoms and Seeking Help

Common Symptoms of Endometriosis

Endometriosis presents a variety of symptoms, with pelvic pain being the most common. This pain often intensifies during menstruation but can also occur at other times, such as during ovulation or intercourse. Other symptoms may include heavy menstrual bleeding, fatigue, and gastrointestinal issues like bloating or diarrhea. Recognizing these symptoms early can aid in timely management and intervention.

Additionally, some women may experience infertility, as endometriosis can affect the reproductive organs. Symptoms can significantly impact daily life, making it essential for individuals to be aware of how endometriosis manifests. Keeping a symptom journal can help track patterns and severity, providing valuable insights when consulting a healthcare provider.

How Symptoms Can Vary Among Individuals

Each woman's experience with endometriosis can differ greatly, influenced by factors such as genetics, hormonal levels, and overall health. While some women may have mild symptoms but severe endometriosis, others may experience debilitating pain with minimal physical findings. This variability makes it crucial for women to be proactive in understanding their bodies and how symptoms may differ from those of others.

Recognizing that endometriosis is not a one-size-fits-all condition can empower women to advocate for themselves. Keeping a detailed account of individual symptoms, triggers, and responses to treatment can assist healthcare providers in tailoring effective management strategies.

When to See a Healthcare Professional

If you experience persistent pelvic pain, painful periods, or other concerning symptoms, it's important to consult a healthcare professional. Early intervention can prevent complications and improve the quality of life. Don't hesitate to seek help if symptoms interfere with daily activities or lead to distress; acknowledging the need for professional support is a vital step in managing endometriosis.

A healthcare professional can provide an assessment and guide you through the next steps, which may include referrals to specialists or diagnostic testing. It's essential to be proactive about your health and seek support when needed.

Importance of a Comprehensive Evaluation

A comprehensive evaluation is crucial in diagnosing endometriosis, as it involves assessing medical history, symptoms, and a physical examination. This thorough approach ensures that other conditions with similar symptoms are ruled out. The more information the healthcare provider has, the better they can recommend an appropriate course of action.

In addition to a physical examination, a comprehensive evaluation may include imaging studies, such as ultrasounds or MRIs, to identify the presence and extent of endometrial tissue outside the uterus. This comprehensive approach allows for a more accurate diagnosis and a better understanding of individual needs.

The Role of a Gynecologist in Diagnosis

Gynecologists play a pivotal role in diagnosing and managing endometriosis. They specialize in female reproductive health and are trained to identify symptoms and perform necessary examinations. Upon identifying potential endometriosis, they can recommend treatment options tailored to the individual's condition and preferences.

In many cases, the gynecologist will conduct a pelvic exam, order imaging tests, or perform a laparoscopy, which allows direct visualization of endometrial tissue. This specialized knowledge makes gynecologists vital partners in managing endometriosis effectively.

Understanding the Difference Between Normal Menstrual Pain and Endometriosis Pain

Distinguishing between normal menstrual pain and pain caused by endometriosis is essential for timely intervention. Normal menstrual cramps typically involve mild to moderate pain, while endometriosis pain is often more severe, persistent, and may not improve with over-the-counter pain relievers. This distinction can guide women in seeking appropriate medical advice.

Recognizing the characteristics of endometriosis pain can lead to earlier diagnosis and treatment. Women should pay attention to the intensity, duration, and triggers of their pain, as this information can be vital during medical consultations.

Utilizing Pain Diaries to Track Symptoms

Keeping a pain diary can be an effective strategy for managing endometriosis. This tool helps track the frequency, intensity, and nature of pain, alongside other symptoms such as mood and dietary habits. By consistently documenting experiences, women can identify patterns that may correlate with their symptoms, aiding discussions with healthcare providers.

A pain diary can also reveal the effectiveness of different treatments or lifestyle changes over time. This comprehensive documentation can empower women to make informed decisions about their healthcare and advocate for the support they need.

Importance of Open Communication with Doctors

Open communication with healthcare providers is essential for effective endometriosis management. Discussing symptoms candidly, including their impact on daily life and emotional well-being, allows for a more tailored treatment approach. Women should feel comfortable sharing any concerns or questions that arise during their care.

Establishing a trusting relationship with doctors encourages transparency, ensuring that individuals receive comprehensive support and the most suitable treatment options. This dialogue can significantly enhance the quality of care provided.

Referrals to Specialists

In some cases, a referral to a specialist may be necessary for comprehensive endometriosis management. Specialists, such as reproductive endocrinologists or pain management experts, bring specific knowledge and skills that can enhance treatment outcomes. Consulting with a specialist may be particularly beneficial when standard treatments are ineffective or if infertility is a concern.

Healthcare providers can help facilitate these referrals, ensuring that patients receive the specialized care they need. Seeking expert opinions can lead to better management strategies and improved quality of life for those affected by endometriosis.

Second Opinions: When and Why to Seek Them

Seeking a second opinion can be a crucial step if there are uncertainties about a diagnosis or treatment plan for endometriosis. It is particularly important when faced with complex symptoms or when initial treatments do not yield satisfactory results. A fresh perspective can provide new insights or alternative treatment options that may be more effective.

Many women find that a second opinion helps them feel more confident in their treatment choices. Healthcare providers typically understand and encourage patients to seek additional consultations if they feel uncertain, which is an essential aspect of patient empowerment.

Questions to Ask Your Doctor

When visiting a healthcare professional, it's beneficial to come prepared with questions. Inquiring about the nature of endometriosis, available treatment options, potential side effects, and lifestyle modifications can help clarify the management process. Questions can empower patients, allowing them to participate actively in their care.

Additionally, asking about support resources, such as counseling or support groups, can provide emotional backing during the treatment journey. Engaging in this dialogue fosters a collaborative relationship between the patient and provider, enhancing overall care.

Diagnostic Tests Commonly Used

Diagnostic tests are essential for confirming endometriosis and understanding its severity. Common tests include ultrasounds, MRIs, and laparoscopy, each providing different insights into the presence of endometrial tissue. These tests help identify the location and extent of the condition, informing treatment decisions.

Laparoscopy, a minimally invasive surgical procedure, allows doctors to directly visualize and possibly remove endometriosis lesions. Understanding these tests can alleviate anxiety and help patients feel more informed about the diagnostic process.

Support Networks for Women Experiencing Symptoms

Joining support networks can provide emotional relief and practical advice for women dealing with endometriosis. These groups, whether online or in-person, offer a safe space to share experiences and coping strategies. Connecting with others facing similar challenges can create a sense of community and reduce feelings of isolation.

Support networks often provide valuable resources, including information about local healthcare providers, educational materials, and tips for managing symptoms. Engaging with these networks empowers women by fostering a supportive environment and enhancing their overall well-being.

CHAPTER 3:

Pain Management Strategies

Overview of Pain Management Options

Managing pain associated with endometriosis involves a multifaceted approach. The first step is to consult with a healthcare provider who can assess the severity of symptoms and recommend appropriate strategies. Common options include medications, lifestyle adjustments, and alternative therapies tailored to individual needs. Understanding various methods can empower women to take charge of their health and alleviate discomfort.

Pain management strategies can be broadly categorized into pharmacological and non-pharmacological methods. Finding the right balance is essential, as individual responses to treatment can vary widely. Engaging in open discussions with healthcare providers about pain relief options is crucial for developing an effective pain management plan.

Over-the-Counter Pain Relief Medications

Over-the-counter (OTC) pain relief medications, such as ibuprofen and acetaminophen, can provide effective relief for endometriosis-related pain. These medications work by reducing inflammation and blocking pain signals to the brain. It's essential to follow the recommended dosage instructions and to take them with food to minimize gastrointestinal side effects.

For women experiencing mild to moderate pain, OTC medications can be a convenient first-line treatment. However, if pain persists or worsens, it may be time to consult a healthcare provider for further evaluation and more potent options.

Prescription Medications for Endometriosis

For those whose pain is not adequately managed with OTC medications, healthcare providers may prescribe stronger pain relief options. Prescription medications often include nonsteroidal anti-inflammatory drugs (NSAIDs) or stronger opioids for short-term use. It's crucial to discuss the potential side effects and risks associated with these medications, particularly opioids, which can lead to dependence.

In addition to pain relievers, prescription medications can also help manage the hormonal aspects of endometriosis. This might include hormonal contraceptives, which can reduce menstrual flow and alleviate pain, thus improving quality of life.

Hormonal Treatments and Their Benefits

Hormonal treatments play a significant role in managing endometriosis symptoms by regulating the menstrual cycle and reducing the growth of endometrial tissue. Options include birth control pills, hormonal IUDs, and GnRH agonists, which can induce a temporary menopause-like state, lowering estrogen levels and subsequently reducing pain.

Discussing the potential benefits and side effects of hormonal treatments with a healthcare provider is essential for making informed decisions. These treatments can offer significant relief, but they may not be suitable for everyone, highlighting the need for personalized care.

Non-Pharmacological Pain Management Techniques

Non-pharmacological techniques, such as heat therapy, TENS (transcutaneous electrical nerve stimulation), and massage, can be effective for managing endometriosis-related pain. Heat therapy, for instance, can relax muscles and reduce cramping, while TENS can help block pain signals through electrical stimulation.

Incorporating these techniques into daily routines can provide additional relief and complement medication. Women are encouraged to explore various non-drug approaches to find what works best for their individual pain management plans.

Physical Therapy and Its Role

Physical therapy can be a valuable resource for women with endometriosis, focusing on pelvic floor therapy to address muscle tension and pain. A qualified physical therapist can create a personalized treatment plan that may include stretching, strengthening exercises, and manual therapy to alleviate discomfort.

Regular sessions can help improve mobility and reduce pain, providing women with practical tools to manage their symptoms more effectively. Women should seek out therapists with experience in treating pelvic pain to ensure they receive the best care.

Lifestyle Changes to Help Reduce Pain

Making lifestyle changes can significantly impact pain levels associated with endometriosis. This includes adopting a balanced diet rich in anti-inflammatory foods, maintaining a healthy weight, and managing stress effectively. Keeping a symptom diary can also help identify triggers and develop coping strategies.

Incorporating healthy habits, such as staying hydrated, prioritizing sleep, and reducing caffeine and alcohol intake, can lead to better overall well-being. These changes empower women to take proactive steps in managing their condition.

Mindfulness and Relaxation Techniques

Mindfulness and relaxation techniques, such as deep breathing, meditation, and yoga, can help alleviate the psychological and physical stress associated with endometriosis. Practicing mindfulness allows individuals to stay present and manage pain without becoming overwhelmed.

Implementing these techniques regularly can lead to reduced anxiety and improved emotional well-being. Women are encouraged to explore different practices to find what resonates with them and incorporate it into their daily routine.

Importance of Exercise and Movement

Regular physical activity is essential for managing endometriosis symptoms, as it can reduce inflammation, improve circulation, and enhance overall mood. Low-impact exercises, such as walking, swimming, or cycling, are excellent options for those experiencing pain.

Creating a consistent exercise routine can lead to long-term benefits, including better pain management and improved quality of life. Women should consult with a healthcare provider or physical therapist to design an exercise program that suits their individual capabilities.

Nutritional Considerations for Pain Management

Nutrition plays a pivotal role in managing endometriosis-related pain. A diet rich in fruits, vegetables, whole grains, and omega-3 fatty acids can help reduce inflammation. Women are encouraged to limit processed foods, sugar, and saturated fats, which can exacerbate symptoms.

Incorporating specific foods, such as leafy greens and fatty fish, can provide essential nutrients that support overall health. Consulting a registered dietitian can help tailor dietary choices to individual needs and preferences.

Alternative Therapies (Acupuncture, Chiropractic Care)

Alternative therapies, including acupuncture and chiropractic care, can offer additional support for managing endometriosis symptoms. Acupuncture has been shown to help reduce pain and regulate menstrual cycles, while chiropractic adjustments can improve spinal alignment and relieve discomfort.

Seeking practitioners who specialize in these therapies can enhance treatment outcomes. Women should communicate openly with their healthcare providers about any alternative therapies they are considering to ensure they complement existing treatments.

Support Groups and Counseling Options

Joining support groups or seeking counseling can provide emotional support and practical advice for managing endometriosis. Sharing experiences with others who understand the challenges can help reduce feelings of isolation and provide coping strategies.

Counseling, whether individual or group-based, can assist in addressing the emotional toll of living with a chronic condition. Women are encouraged to explore these resources for additional support and guidance.

Importance of Individualized Pain Management Plans

Creating an individualized pain management plan is essential for effectively addressing endometriosis symptoms. This plan should consider a woman's specific symptoms, medical history, and lifestyle factors. Regular check-ins with healthcare providers can help adjust the plan as needed.

Women should actively participate in their pain management discussions, expressing their preferences and concerns to ensure that their needs are met. An individualized approach can lead to more effective management and improved quality of life.

CHAPTER 4:

Fertility and Endometriosis

Connection between Endometriosis and Fertility Issues

Endometriosis can significantly impact fertility due to the presence of endometrial-like tissue outside the uterus, which can cause scarring and adhesions in the reproductive organs. These changes can lead to blocked fallopian tubes, which are essential for sperm and egg transport, as well as altered hormonal balance that can affect ovulation. Understanding this connection is crucial for women with endometriosis who are trying to conceive, as it may require specific management strategies to improve their chances of pregnancy.

The severity of endometriosis varies among individuals, with some experiencing mild symptoms while others face severe complications that can hinder fertility. Therefore, women diagnosed with endometriosis should consult healthcare providers to assess the extent of their condition and its potential impact on fertility. This connection underscores the importance of early diagnosis and tailored treatment plans to enhance reproductive outcomes.

How Endometriosis Can Affect Ovulation and Implantation

Endometriosis can disrupt the normal hormonal environment necessary for ovulation by causing inflammation and hormone imbalances in the body. This disruption can lead to irregular menstrual cycles and anovulation (the absence of ovulation), making it challenging for women to conceive. Additionally, the presence of endometrial tissue can interfere with the implantation of a fertilized egg in the uterus, further complicating the conception process.

To understand how endometriosis affects ovulation and implantation, women should track their menstrual cycles and any associated symptoms, such as pelvic pain or irregular periods. Working closely with a healthcare provider can help identify these issues and explore treatment options that support ovulation and improve the chances of successful implantation.

Fertility Tests and Assessments for Women with Endometriosis

Women with endometriosis should undergo a comprehensive evaluation to assess their fertility status. This typically includes a pelvic exam, imaging tests like ultrasound or MRI, and blood tests to evaluate hormone levels. A hysterosalpingogram (HSG) may also be performed to check for blockages in the fallopian tubes, which is crucial for determining the most effective treatment options.

By conducting these assessments, healthcare providers can identify specific fertility issues related to endometriosis. This information allows for personalized treatment plans tailored to the individual's needs, ultimately providing a clearer path forward in their journey to conceive.

Treatment Options for Improving Fertility

Treatment options for improving fertility in women with endometriosis can vary widely based on the severity of the condition and the individual's reproductive goals. Common options include hormonal therapies to reduce the growth of endometrial tissue and surgical interventions to remove adhesions or endometriosis lesions. These treatments aim to create a more favorable environment for conception.

In addition to traditional treatments, lifestyle changes such as maintaining a healthy diet, regular exercise, and managing stress can also support fertility. Women should discuss these options with their healthcare provider to develop a holistic approach that aligns with their fertility goals.

Role of Assisted Reproductive Technologies (ART)

Assisted reproductive technologies (ART) play a crucial role in helping women with endometriosis conceive when traditional methods are unsuccessful. Techniques such as in vitro fertilization (IVF) can bypass some of the challenges posed by endometriosis, as eggs are retrieved and fertilized outside the body before being implanted into the uterus. This process allows for better control over timing and increases the chances of pregnancy.

Women considering ART should consult with a fertility specialist who can provide insights into the best approach for their specific situation. Understanding the benefits and potential risks associated with ART can empower women to make informed decisions regarding their fertility treatment options.

Importance of Working with a Fertility Specialist

Working with a fertility specialist is essential for women with endometriosis who are seeking to conceive. These experts possess the knowledge and experience to navigate the complexities of endometriosis and its impact on fertility. They can provide personalized treatment plans, recommend appropriate tests, and guide women through the various fertility treatment options available.

By collaborating closely with a fertility specialist, women can gain access to advanced diagnostic tools and innovative treatment approaches tailored to their unique needs. This partnership can significantly enhance the chances of achieving a successful pregnancy.

Emotional Considerations Regarding Fertility and Endometriosis

The emotional toll of navigating fertility challenges can be significant for women with endometriosis. Feelings of frustration, sadness, and anxiety may arise as they confront the difficulties associated with both their condition and the desire to conceive. It's essential for women to acknowledge these emotions and seek support from friends, family, or mental health professionals.

Participating in support groups or therapy can provide a safe space to express feelings and connect with others facing similar challenges. This emotional support can be vital in managing stress and maintaining a positive outlook throughout the fertility journey.

Options for Preserving Fertility

For women diagnosed with endometriosis, considering options for preserving fertility is important, especially if they are not ready to conceive immediately. One approach is egg freezing, where eggs are harvested and frozen for future use, allowing women to maintain their reproductive options despite the progression of endometriosis. This option can be particularly valuable for younger women who wish to delay pregnancy.

Another option is to explore hormonal treatments that can suppress the growth of endometrial tissue while preserving ovarian function. Consulting with a fertility specialist can help women understand these preservation methods and make informed decisions based on their personal circumstances and future family planning goals.

Exploring Surrogacy and Adoption

For some women with endometriosis, surrogacy or adoption may be viable alternatives if they encounter ongoing fertility challenges. Surrogacy involves another woman carrying a pregnancy for those unable to conceive due to medical issues. This option allows individuals to experience parenthood without the physical challenges of pregnancy.

Adoption offers a path to parenthood that can be equally fulfilling. Women considering these options should research and connect with professionals experienced in surrogacy or adoption processes to ensure a smooth journey. Understanding legal requirements, emotional implications, and available resources can help women navigate these complex decisions.

Support Resources for Women Facing Fertility Challenges

Various support resources are available for women facing fertility challenges related to endometriosis. Support groups, both in-person and online, provide a platform for sharing experiences, exchanging advice, and receiving encouragement from others in similar situations. Additionally, fertility clinics often offer counseling services to help women cope with the emotional aspects of their journey.

Women can also benefit from educational resources, including books, webinars, and workshops focused on fertility and endometriosis. Engaging with these resources can empower women with knowledge and connections to better navigate their fertility challenges.

Common Misconceptions about Endometriosis and Fertility

There are many misconceptions surrounding endometriosis and its impact on fertility. One common myth is that all women with endometriosis will experience infertility, which is not true. While endometriosis can affect fertility, many women still conceive naturally or with treatment. Understanding the nuances of this condition is vital for managing expectations and reducing anxiety.

Addressing these misconceptions can empower women to seek appropriate care and support. Open conversations with healthcare providers can help clarify any doubts and provide accurate information regarding the relationship between endometriosis and fertility.

Success Stories and Testimonials

Listening to success stories and testimonials from women who have navigated the challenges of endometriosis and achieved pregnancy can be inspiring and encouraging. These stories often highlight the diverse paths taken, whether through medical treatment, lifestyle changes, or alternative approaches like adoption. Hearing about the experiences of others can foster hope and resilience among women facing similar struggles.

Sharing these success stories through forums, social media, or support groups can create a sense of community and solidarity. Women should feel empowered to share their journeys, as their stories may help uplift and motivate others in their pursuit of motherhood.

Importance of a Supportive Partner

Having a supportive partner during the journey of dealing with endometriosis and fertility challenges is invaluable. Emotional support from a partner can significantly alleviate stress and anxiety, fostering a sense of teamwork in navigating the complexities of treatment options and decision-making. Open communication is essential, allowing both partners to express their feelings, concerns, and hopes.

Additionally, partners can participate in medical appointments and support group meetings, enhancing their understanding of the challenges faced. This involvement can strengthen the bond between partners and create a nurturing environment conducive to facing fertility challenges together.

CHAPTER 5:

Surgical Treatment Options

Overview of Surgical Options for Endometriosis

Surgical options for endometriosis aim to remove or reduce endometrial tissue and alleviate symptoms. The primary goal of surgery is to relieve pain, improve quality of life, and enhance fertility. Understanding the available surgical procedures can help you make informed decisions about your treatment options.

There are two main types of surgery for endometriosis: laparoscopy, a minimally invasive procedure where small incisions are made, and laparotomy, which involves a larger abdominal incision. Laparoscopy typically offers quicker recovery and less postoperative pain, making it a popular choice for many patients. However, the choice of procedure depends on the severity of endometriosis, its location, and your specific health needs.

Types of Surgery Available (Laparoscopy, Laparotomy)

Laparoscopy is performed using a laparoscope, a thin tube with a camera, which allows the surgeon to visualize and treat endometrial lesions through small incisions. This technique often results in shorter hospital stays and faster recovery times compared to traditional surgeries. Patients usually experience less pain and scarring, making it an appealing option for many.

Laparotomy, on the other hand, may be necessary for more extensive cases of endometriosis, where larger lesions are present or when the surgeon needs to access deep-seated tissue. This approach allows for a more comprehensive assessment and treatment but requires a longer recovery period. It's crucial to discuss the pros and cons of each type with your healthcare provider to determine the best approach for your situation.

Indications for Surgery

Surgery for endometriosis is typically indicated when other treatments, such as medication or lifestyle changes, have failed to provide adequate relief. Common reasons include severe pelvic pain, pain during intercourse, infertility, or large endometriosis cysts (endometriomas). Your doctor will evaluate your symptoms and the extent of your endometriosis to determine if surgery is the right option.

In some cases, surgery may also be recommended for diagnostic purposes, particularly if imaging tests have not provided clear answers. It's essential to have open discussions with your healthcare team about your symptoms and treatment goals to assess whether surgery is necessary for you.

What to Expect Before, During, and After Surgery

Before surgery, your healthcare provider will provide detailed instructions, which may include dietary restrictions and medication adjustments. It's common to undergo preoperative tests, such as blood tests or imaging studies, to ensure you're fit for the procedure. You should also prepare for recovery by arranging for help at home, as you may need assistance in the days following surgery.

During the surgery, anesthesia will be administered, and the procedure's length will vary based on complexity. Afterward, you'll be monitored in a recovery area before being sent home, usually the same day or the next. Expect some discomfort and fatigue in the initial days post-surgery, and be prepared to follow your surgeon's guidelines for care to ensure a smooth recovery.

Potential Risks and Complications

As with any surgical procedure, there are potential risks and complications associated with surgery for endometriosis. Common risks include infection, bleeding, and reactions to anesthesia. Specific complications can involve damage to surrounding organs, such as the bladder or intestines, especially in more complex cases of endometriosis.

It's essential to discuss these risks with your surgeon before the procedure. Understanding the potential complications can help you make an informed decision and prepare for your surgery and recovery.

Importance of Selecting a Skilled Surgeon

Choosing a skilled surgeon is critical for successful endometriosis surgery. A surgeon with experience in treating endometriosis will have a better understanding of the condition and its complications, which can lead to more effective treatment outcomes. It's advisable to seek a surgeon who specializes in minimally invasive techniques, as these often result in less postoperative pain and faster recovery.

When selecting a surgeon, consider their credentials, experience, and patient reviews. Don't hesitate to ask for referrals from your healthcare provider or other patients. Trust and communication with your surgeon can significantly influence your surgical experience and recovery process.

Post-Surgery Recovery Tips

Post-surgery recovery involves following your surgeon's instructions closely to facilitate healing. Rest is crucial in the initial days following surgery; avoid strenuous activities and heavy lifting. Applying heat to the abdomen can help alleviate discomfort, while over-the-counter pain relievers may be recommended to manage pain.

Stay hydrated and focus on nutritious foods to support your body's healing process. If you experience severe pain, fever, or other concerning symptoms, contact your healthcare provider immediately for further evaluation.

Impact of Surgery on Fertility

Surgery for endometriosis can have a significant impact on fertility, often improving the chances of conception. By removing endometrial lesions and scar tissue, surgery can restore normal anatomy and function of reproductive organs. Many women find that their pain is reduced post-surgery, which can facilitate attempts to conceive.

However, it's important to have realistic expectations, as not all women will achieve pregnancy following surgery. Discuss fertility goals with your healthcare provider before surgery to explore additional treatments, such as in vitro fertilization (IVF), if needed.

Monitoring for Recurrence after Surgery

Monitoring for recurrence after endometriosis surgery is essential, as the condition can return. Your healthcare provider may recommend regular follow-ups, including pelvic exams and imaging studies, to assess for any signs of recurrent endometriosis. Being proactive can help manage symptoms and address issues early.

It's also beneficial to keep track of any symptoms you experience post-surgery, as this information can guide discussions with your healthcare provider. Being vigilant about your health can aid in effective long-term management of endometriosis.

Long-Term Management Post-Surgery

Long-term management of endometriosis involves a multifaceted approach, including medication, lifestyle changes, and regular follow-ups. Hormonal treatments, such as birth control pills, can help manage symptoms and reduce the risk of recurrence. Incorporating a balanced diet, regular exercise, and stress management techniques can also play a significant role in overall health.

Engaging in support groups or therapy can be beneficial for emotional well-being, as managing a chronic condition can be challenging. Your healthcare provider can help you develop a comprehensive management plan tailored to your needs.

Importance of Follow-Up Care

Follow-up care after endometriosis surgery is crucial for monitoring recovery and preventing complications. Schedule follow-up appointments as recommended by your surgeon, typically within a few weeks post-surgery.

During these visits, your doctor will assess your recovery, address any concerns, and adjust your treatment plan as needed.

Maintaining open communication with your healthcare team is vital to ensure you receive the best care possible. Discuss any new or lingering symptoms and seek guidance on lifestyle changes or additional treatments that may enhance your recovery and overall health.

Support Groups for Post-Surgery Patients

Support groups can provide invaluable resources and emotional support for individuals recovering from endometriosis surgery. Connecting with others who share similar experiences can help you feel less isolated and provide insights into managing symptoms and navigating recovery challenges.

You can find support groups through local healthcare facilities, online platforms, or organizations dedicated to endometriosis awareness. Participating in these groups can also empower you with information, coping strategies, and encouragement during your healing journey.

Questions to Ask Your Surgeon

When preparing for surgery, it's essential to have a list of questions for your surgeon to clarify any concerns and ensure you understand the process. Inquire about the specific surgical procedure, recovery expectations, potential risks, and how the surgery may impact your symptoms and fertility.

Additionally, asking about follow-up care, lifestyle changes post-surgery, and resources for support can enhance your understanding and prepare you for the journey ahead. A well-informed patient is better equipped to make decisions that align with their health goals and needs.

CHAPTER 6:

Nutrition and Lifestyle Modifications

Role of Diet in Managing Endometriosis Symptoms

Diet plays a crucial role in managing endometriosis symptoms, as certain foods can either exacerbate or alleviate pain and discomfort. A balanced diet rich in whole foods, such as fruits, vegetables, whole grains, and lean proteins, can help reduce inflammation and support overall health. It's essential to focus on nutrient-dense options that nourish the body and may alleviate some symptoms associated with endometriosis.

To effectively manage endometriosis through diet, start by identifying foods that trigger your symptoms. Keeping a food diary can help you track your meals and symptoms, making it easier to pinpoint specific foods that may be causing discomfort. This awareness allows for more informed dietary choices that can lead to improved symptom management.

Anti-inflammatory Foods to Include

Incorporating anti-inflammatory foods into your diet can significantly benefit those managing endometriosis. Foods such as fatty fish (like salmon and sardines), leafy greens, berries, nuts, and seeds contain nutrients that help combat inflammation. Omega-3 fatty acids found in fish and flaxseeds are particularly effective in reducing inflammation and pain.

To make anti-inflammatory foods a staple in your diet, aim for at least two servings of fatty fish per week and incorporate a variety of colorful fruits and vegetables into your meals. Preparing meals with olive oil, turmeric, and ginger can also enhance flavor while providing additional anti-inflammatory benefits.

Foods to Avoid with Endometriosis

Certain foods may worsen endometriosis symptoms and should be avoided to help manage the condition effectively. Common culprits include processed foods, high-sugar items, trans fats, and refined carbohydrates, which can contribute to inflammation and hormonal imbalance. Dairy products may also trigger symptoms in some individuals, so it's advisable to assess your body's reaction.

To minimize these foods in your diet, focus on whole, unprocessed options. Cooking at home allows you to control ingredients and avoid hidden additives that can exacerbate symptoms. Read food labels carefully and choose products that are lower in sugar and free from unhealthy fats.

Importance of Hydration

Staying adequately hydrated is vital for managing endometriosis symptoms, as hydration can help reduce bloating and support overall bodily functions. Drinking plenty of water throughout the day aids digestion and helps maintain energy levels. Aim for at least eight glasses of water daily, and increase your intake if you engage in physical activity or live in a hot climate.

To enhance hydration, consider including hydrating foods such as cucumbers, watermelon, and oranges in your diet. Herbal teas, especially those with anti-inflammatory properties like chamomile or ginger, can also be a soothing addition to your hydration routine.

Nutritional Supplements to Consider

Nutritional supplements can provide additional support for managing endometriosis symptoms. Omega-3 fatty acids, vitamin D, and magnesium are commonly recommended supplements that may help alleviate inflammation, improve mood, and promote overall well-being. However, it's important to consult with a healthcare provider before starting any new supplements to determine the appropriate dosages for your specific needs.

Incorporating supplements into your routine can be as simple as taking them with meals to improve absorption. Keep a schedule or set reminders to ensure consistency. Working with a nutritionist can also help tailor a supplement plan that complements your dietary choices.

Impact of Caffeine and Alcohol on Symptoms

Caffeine and alcohol can have varying effects on endometriosis symptoms. Some studies suggest that caffeine may contribute to increased pain and inflammation, while alcohol can exacerbate bloating and hormonal fluctuations. Monitoring your intake of these substances can help you identify any correlations between consumption and symptom severity.

To manage symptoms effectively, consider reducing or eliminating caffeine and alcohol from your diet. Opt for caffeine-free herbal teas and sparkling water instead of alcohol. Pay attention to how your body responds, and adjust your consumption accordingly to find what works best for you.

Exercise Recommendations and Benefits

Regular exercise can provide significant benefits for those with endometriosis, including reduced pain, improved mood, and enhanced overall well-being. Activities like walking, yoga, and swimming can help alleviate discomfort while promoting relaxation and stress relief. Aim for at least 30 minutes of moderate exercise most days of the week to experience the positive effects on your symptoms.

Incorporating a variety of activities into your routine can keep exercise enjoyable and engaging. Consider joining a class or finding a workout buddy for motivation. Listen to your body and adjust the intensity and type of exercise based on how you feel to avoid overexertion.

Importance of Sleep and Stress Management

Sleep and stress management are crucial for individuals managing endometriosis symptoms. Quality sleep helps the body repair itself and manage pain levels, while effective stress management techniques can help reduce the overall burden of symptoms. Aim for 7-9 hours of restorative sleep each night and establish a calming bedtime routine.

Incorporate stress-reducing practices such as meditation, deep breathing exercises, or gentle yoga into your daily routine. Finding activities that promote relaxation and balance can significantly impact your overall well-being, leading to a more manageable experience with endometriosis symptoms.

Building a Supportive Social Network

Having a supportive social network is essential for individuals dealing with endometriosis. Connecting with friends, family, or support groups can provide emotional support, shared experiences, and practical advice for managing the condition. Don't hesitate to reach out and communicate your needs to those around you.

To build your network, consider joining local or online support groups focused on endometriosis. Sharing your experiences with others who understand can help reduce feelings of isolation. Engaging in social activities that bring joy can also help foster connections and provide a positive outlet.

Incorporating Relaxation Techniques into Daily Life

Incorporating relaxation techniques into your daily life can greatly benefit those managing endometriosis. Practices such as mindfulness, meditation, and deep breathing can help alleviate stress and promote a sense of calm. Set aside a few minutes each day to practice these techniques, creating a space where you can unwind and focus on your well-being.

To get started, find a quiet space where you can sit comfortably. Use guided meditation apps or videos to help you learn different relaxation techniques. Even brief moments of mindfulness throughout your day can help reduce anxiety and improve your overall mental health.

Tips for Maintaining a Healthy Weight

Maintaining a healthy weight can positively influence endometriosis symptoms and overall health. Excess body weight can increase inflammation and hormonal imbalances, potentially worsening symptoms. To achieve and maintain a healthy weight, focus on a balanced diet and regular physical activity tailored to your needs and preferences.

To effectively manage your weight, track your food intake and physical activity using apps or journals. Set realistic goals and celebrate small victories along the way. Working with a nutritionist can provide personalized guidance and strategies to support your weight management journey.

Mindful Eating Practices

Mindful eating practices can enhance your relationship with food while supporting symptom management for endometriosis. This approach encourages individuals to focus on their food choices, savor each bite, and listen to their body's hunger cues. By practicing mindfulness during meals, you can develop a greater awareness of how certain foods impact your symptoms.

To practice mindful eating, start by eliminating distractions during meals, such as screens or multitasking. Take the time to appreciate the colors, flavors, and textures of your food. Chewing slowly and paying attention to your body's signals can help you feel more satisfied and prevent overeating.

Resources for Meal Planning and Recipes

Accessing resources for meal planning and recipes can simplify managing endometriosis through diet. Look for cookbooks, websites, and apps that focus on anti-inflammatory or endometriosis-friendly recipes. These resources can provide inspiration and help you create balanced meal plans tailored to your dietary needs.

To streamline your meal planning process, consider setting aside time each week to plan meals and create a shopping list. Batch cooking or preparing meals in advance can save time during busy weeks, ensuring you always have nutritious options on hand. Engage with online communities for additional support and recipe ideas that suit your lifestyle.

CHAPTER 7:

Emotional and Psychological Support

Understanding the Emotional Impact of Endometriosis

Endometriosis can significantly affect a woman's emotional well-being, leading to feelings of isolation, frustration, and sadness. The chronic pain and unpredictable nature of the condition can disrupt daily life, impacting work, relationships, and social activities. Recognizing these emotional challenges is the first step toward effective management. It's important to acknowledge feelings and understand that emotional responses are valid and common among those with endometriosis.

Women experiencing endometriosis may benefit from professional guidance to navigate these emotional hurdles. Supportive environments and open discussions about feelings can foster better coping mechanisms.

Taking proactive steps toward understanding and addressing emotional challenges can help in the overall management of the condition, empowering women to take control of their health.

Importance of Mental Health Care

Mental health care is a crucial aspect of managing endometriosis, as the stress and pain can lead to anxiety and depression. Seeking help from mental health professionals can provide valuable tools to cope with emotional distress. Cognitive-behavioral therapy (CBT) and other therapeutic approaches can help identify and alter negative thought patterns, fostering a more positive mindset and enhancing resilience against the challenges posed by endometriosis.

Integrating mental health care into the treatment plan also emphasizes the importance of self-compassion and emotional awareness. Regular check-ins with a therapist or counselor can aid in maintaining mental well-being, helping individuals manage their symptoms more effectively while addressing any psychological burdens that arise from living with endometriosis.

Counseling Options for Emotional Support

Counseling offers a structured environment for women to discuss the emotional impact of endometriosis. Trained therapists can help identify feelings of anxiety, depression, or frustration, providing coping strategies tailored to individual needs. Various types of counseling, such as individual therapy, group therapy, or couples counseling, can be beneficial depending on personal preferences and circumstances.

Engaging in counseling can provide a sense of relief, as it allows for the exploration of feelings in a safe space. It can also foster a deeper understanding of the condition, equipping women with the tools necessary to articulate their experiences and advocate for their needs within their personal and professional lives.

Mindfulness and Stress Reduction Techniques

Mindfulness practices can play a significant role in managing the emotional and physical symptoms of endometriosis. Techniques such as meditation, deep breathing, and yoga help create a state of relaxation, reducing stress and promoting emotional balance. Incorporating these practices into a daily routine can empower women to take control of their mental health and reduce the intensity of pain and discomfort.

To begin, set aside a few minutes each day to practice mindfulness. Simple activities like focusing on breath, engaging in guided meditation, or stretching can make a difference in how you respond to stressors. Regular practice can cultivate a greater sense of calm, helping women cope more effectively with the challenges of endometriosis.

Building a Support System (Friends, Family, Support Groups)

Establishing a support system is essential for managing the emotional toll of endometriosis. Friends and family members can provide love and encouragement, while support groups offer shared experiences and practical advice. Connecting with others who understand the journey can alleviate feelings of isolation and provide comfort during difficult times.

To build a support network, reach out to friends and family and share your experiences. Additionally, consider joining local or online support groups where you can connect with others facing similar challenges. This community can offer invaluable insights, emotional support, and practical tips for navigating life with endometriosis.

Navigating Relationships and Intimacy with Endometriosis

Endometriosis can impact relationships and intimacy, often causing anxiety and strain. Open communication with partners is vital for navigating these challenges. Discussing feelings, fears, and the physical limitations caused by endometriosis can foster understanding and strengthen the relationship.

When intimacy is affected, exploring alternative ways to connect—such as emotional closeness, non-sexual affection, or engaging in shared activities—can help maintain a strong bond. Setting boundaries and discussing needs with partners can lead to a more supportive and fulfilling relationship, ultimately benefiting both parties involved.

Resources for Self-Care and Wellness

Self-care is a fundamental aspect of managing endometriosis, encompassing physical, emotional, and mental well-being. Creating a personalized self-care routine can include activities such as exercise, healthy eating, adequate rest, and hobbies that promote relaxation and joy. It's essential to listen to your body and adjust your activities based on what feels best.

Explore various self-care resources such as books, online courses, or wellness apps that focus on mindfulness, nutrition, or exercise tailored for those with endometriosis. Regularly engaging in self-care practices not only enhances physical health but also contributes to emotional resilience, allowing women to better cope with the challenges of endometriosis.

Importance of Expressing Feelings and Seeking Help

Expressing feelings is crucial for emotional health, especially when dealing with a condition like endometriosis. Journaling, talking to trusted friends, or engaging in creative outlets can provide a means to articulate emotions and thoughts. Acknowledging and voicing feelings can prevent them from becoming overwhelming and can foster a sense of relief.

Seeking help when needed is equally important. This can involve professional counseling, joining support groups, or discussing feelings with family. Taking the initiative to express emotions and seek support demonstrates strength and commitment to one's emotional well-being, ultimately leading to better management of the condition.

Coping Strategies for Dealing with Stress and Anxiety

Effective coping strategies can significantly alleviate stress and anxiety related to endometriosis. Techniques such as setting realistic goals, practicing time management, and breaking tasks into smaller steps can help create a sense of accomplishment. Identifying triggers of stress and actively addressing them can lead to a more balanced emotional state.

Incorporating relaxation techniques, such as progressive muscle relaxation or guided imagery, can also be beneficial. These strategies help promote calmness and reduce the physiological symptoms of anxiety, providing women with tools to manage their stress more effectively and maintain a sense of control over their emotional health.

The Role of Journaling and Reflection

Journaling can serve as a powerful tool for managing the emotional challenges of endometriosis. Writing down thoughts, feelings, and experiences provides a safe space for self-expression and can aid in identifying patterns or triggers related to pain and emotional distress. Regular reflection through journaling allows for deeper understanding and insight into one's journey.

To start journaling, set aside a few minutes each day to write freely about your experiences, challenges, and victories. This practice can enhance emotional awareness and help track symptoms, making it easier to communicate with healthcare providers about your condition and its impact on your life.

Finding Empowerment through Advocacy

Advocacy plays a crucial role in managing endometriosis and can provide a sense of empowerment. Understanding your condition, educating yourself about treatment options, and sharing your experiences can help raise awareness and improve access to care. Becoming involved in advocacy efforts—such as joining campaigns or participating in community discussions—can strengthen your voice and foster connections with others in similar situations.

To begin advocating, consider sharing your story through social media, blogs, or local events. Engaging in these activities not only benefits personal growth but also contributes to a broader movement aimed at increasing awareness and improving support for those affected by endometriosis.

Importance of Maintaining Hobbies and Interests

Engaging in hobbies and interests can provide a vital outlet for emotional expression and stress relief for women with endometriosis. Maintaining activities that bring joy and fulfillment helps create a sense of normalcy amidst the challenges of managing a chronic condition. Whether it's painting, gardening, or participating in sports, finding time for hobbies can enhance overall well-being.

To incorporate hobbies into your life, schedule regular time for these activities, ensuring they remain a priority despite other commitments. Exploring new interests can also foster a sense of adventure and excitement, helping combat feelings of isolation and frustration commonly associated with endometriosis.

Celebrating Small Victories in Management

Recognizing and celebrating small victories can significantly enhance motivation and emotional resilience in managing endometriosis. Acknowledging achievements, whether related to symptom management, emotional well-being, or daily tasks, reinforces a positive mindset and fosters a sense of accomplishment. Celebrating these milestones can encourage continued commitment to self-care and management strategies.

To effectively celebrate small victories, consider keeping a gratitude journal or sharing accomplishments with friends or family. By creating a culture of positivity and recognition, women can cultivate a supportive environment that empowers them to navigate their endometriosis journey with confidence and resilience.

CHAPTER 8:

The Role of Advocacy and Education

Importance of Patient Advocacy

Patient advocacy is crucial in navigating the complexities of healthcare, especially for those with endometriosis. It empowers patients to take control of their health journey, ensuring their voices are heard and respected in medical settings. By advocating for themselves, individuals can better communicate their symptoms, treatment preferences, and overall healthcare goals, leading to more tailored and effective care.

To practice advocacy, patients can start by educating themselves about endometriosis, its symptoms, and available treatments. Keeping detailed health records and a symptom diary can enhance discussions with healthcare providers. Engaging in open dialogues, asking questions, and expressing concerns are vital steps in advocating for one's needs and rights within the healthcare system.

Understanding Your Rights in Healthcare

Understanding your rights in healthcare is essential for receiving fair treatment and access to necessary medical services. Patients have the right to be informed about their conditions, participate in decisions about their treatment, and receive respectful care without discrimination. Familiarizing yourself with these rights can help you navigate the healthcare system more confidently.

To exercise these rights, start by researching local laws and regulations regarding patient care in your area. Be proactive in discussions with healthcare providers, asking for clarity on any aspect of your treatment plan. Remember, you have the right to seek a second opinion or change providers if you feel your rights are not being upheld.

Engaging with Advocacy Organizations

Engaging with advocacy organizations can provide invaluable support and resources for those affected by endometriosis. These organizations often offer information on treatment options, host support groups, and advocate for policy changes that benefit patients. Connecting with such groups can help patients feel less isolated and more empowered in their health journey.

To get involved, research local and national organizations dedicated to endometriosis awareness. Attend workshops, webinars, and support group meetings to meet others with similar experiences. Many organizations also offer volunteer opportunities, allowing you to contribute to advocacy efforts while gaining knowledge and support.

How to Advocate for Yourself with Healthcare Providers

Advocating for yourself with healthcare providers involves effective communication and preparedness. Start by preparing for appointments with a clear list of symptoms, questions, and any relevant medical history. This will help ensure that you can convey your concerns effectively, making it easier for healthcare providers to understand your situation.

During appointments, don't hesitate to ask questions or request clarifications about your treatment options. It's essential to express your needs and preferences openly, whether it's about pain management, fertility concerns, or lifestyle changes. If you feel your concerns are not being addressed, consider seeking a second opinion from another healthcare provider.

Importance of Raising Awareness about Endometriosis

Raising awareness about endometriosis is vital to improving diagnosis and treatment options for those affected. Many people remain unaware of the condition, leading to delayed diagnoses and inadequate care. By sharing information about endometriosis, you can help educate others and promote a better understanding of the condition.

You can raise awareness through various channels, including social media, community events, and educational workshops. Organizing or participating in campaigns that highlight endometriosis can significantly impact public perception and encourage more individuals to seek help and support for their symptoms.

Educational Resources for Patients and Families

Accessing educational resources is essential for patients and families dealing with endometriosis. Resources such as pamphlets, online articles, and videos can provide valuable insights into the condition, treatment options, and coping strategies. These materials can empower patients to make informed decisions about their healthcare.

To find suitable resources, check reputable websites of healthcare organizations, hospitals, and advocacy groups. Consider attending workshops or seminars that provide expert information on endometriosis, where you can also connect with other patients and families facing similar challenges.

How to Participate in Awareness Campaigns

Participating in awareness campaigns is a great way to contribute to the fight against endometriosis. These campaigns often involve activities like social media promotion, fundraising events, and community outreach. Getting involved helps spread awareness and fosters a sense of community among those affected by the condition.

To participate, look for local or national campaigns focused on endometriosis awareness. You can volunteer your time, share campaign materials on social media, or even organize your own events, such as walks or educational sessions, to engage your community and raise awareness about the condition.

Sharing Your Story: The Power of Personal Narratives

Sharing your personal story can be a powerful tool in raising awareness about endometriosis. Personal narratives humanize the condition, illustrating the challenges individuals face and the importance of timely diagnosis and treatment. By sharing your experiences, you can inspire others to speak out and seek help.

Consider writing a blog, participating in podcasts, or using social media platforms to share your journey. Whether through personal anecdotes or educational content, your voice can resonate with others, fostering a sense of solidarity and encouraging more open discussions about endometriosis

Encouraging Research and Funding for Endometriosis

Encouraging research and funding for endometriosis is crucial for improving treatments and understanding the condition better. Increased funding can lead to more extensive studies that uncover the causes, symptoms, and effective treatment options. As a patient or advocate, your involvement can help drive this change.

You can support research initiatives by donating to organizations focused on endometriosis research or advocating for funding at the local and national levels. Engaging with lawmakers to discuss the importance of endometriosis research can also contribute to greater awareness and resources dedicated to the condition.

Importance of Educating Peers and Communities

Educating peers and communities about endometriosis is essential for fostering understanding and reducing stigma surrounding the condition. Many people are unaware of the symptoms and impact of endometriosis, which can lead to misconceptions and inadequate support for those affected. By sharing knowledge, you can create a more informed and supportive environment.

Host educational workshops, share informational materials, or use social media to spread awareness. Engaging local schools, community centers, and healthcare providers can also help ensure that more people understand endometriosis and its effects, leading to better support for those impacted.

Building a Supportive Online Presence

Building a supportive online presence can be a valuable resource for individuals with endometriosis. Social media platforms and blogs provide a space for sharing experiences, exchanging advice, and connecting with others facing similar challenges. An online community can offer emotional support and practical tips for managing the condition.

To create a supportive presence, share your journey, post informative content, and engage with others in the community. Encourage open discussions, promote positive coping strategies, and celebrate achievements, no matter how small. Your online support can help others feel less alone in their struggles.

Collaborating with Healthcare Professionals for Better Care

Collaboration with healthcare professionals is key to receiving comprehensive care for endometriosis.

Building strong relationships with your healthcare team allows for open communication about symptoms, treatment options, and personal goals. This collaboration ensures a more personalized approach to managing your health.

To foster this collaboration, schedule regular check-ups, maintain open lines of communication, and express any concerns or preferences you may have regarding your care. Involving various specialists, such as gynecologists, nutritionists, and mental health professionals, can also provide a holistic approach to managing endometriosis effectively.

How to Contribute to the Endometriosis Community

Contributing to the endometriosis community can have a significant impact on awareness, support, and research efforts. Your involvement can take many forms, from volunteering with advocacy organizations to participating in local events. Each contribution helps to create a stronger, more informed community.

Start by exploring local support groups, advocacy organizations, and online forums where you can connect with others. Participate in discussions, share your insights, and offer support to those who may be newly diagnosed or seeking guidance. Every action, no matter how small, helps build a more robust community dedicated to understanding and managing endometriosis.

CHAPTER 9:

Living Well with Endometriosis

Developing a Personalized Management Plan

Creating a personalized management plan for endometriosis is crucial for effectively managing symptoms and improving quality of life. Start by working closely with a healthcare provider who understands your specific condition. Discuss your symptoms, lifestyle, and any previous treatments you have tried. Together, you can identify effective strategies that may include medication, physical therapy, dietary changes, or alternative therapies like acupuncture. Document your goals, preferred treatments, and how you will monitor progress over time.

Once your plan is in place, regularly review and adjust it based on your experiences. Keep a journal to track your symptoms, responses to treatments, and any changes in your condition. This will help you recognize patterns and identify which approaches are most beneficial. Remember that endometriosis can be unpredictable; be open to modifying your plan as needed to ensure it remains effective and relevant to your evolving needs.

Importance of Routine Check-ups and Monitoring

Routine check-ups are essential for managing endometriosis effectively. Regular visits to your healthcare provider allow for continuous monitoring of your condition, enabling early detection of any changes or complications. Schedule appointments at least once a year, or more frequently if your symptoms change or worsen. During these visits, discuss your current treatment plan, any new symptoms, and any concerns you may have.

Monitoring your condition also involves tracking symptoms and treatments outside of appointments. Consider using apps or journals to document your experiences, including pain levels, medication effectiveness, and lifestyle changes. This information can provide valuable insights for your healthcare team and help tailor your management plan to better suit your needs.

Adjusting to Changes and Setbacks

Living with endometriosis often involves unexpected changes and setbacks, making adaptability key to managing the condition. It's important to recognize that not every day will be the same; some days may bring increased pain or fatigue. When you encounter a setback, assess your situation calmly. Identify any factors that may have contributed to the change and discuss these with your healthcare provider for potential adjustments to your treatment plan.

Developing coping strategies can also help you navigate these challenges. This might include practicing mindfulness, engaging in gentle exercise, or seeking support from friends or family. Remember, it's normal to feel frustrated, but allow yourself to process these emotions and focus on self-care to regain your balance.

Embracing a Positive Mindset

A positive mindset can significantly impact your experience with endometriosis. Focus on what you can control, such as your daily habits, self-care practices, and support systems. Start each day with affirmations or set intentions to foster a positive outlook. Surround yourself with supportive people who uplift you and understand your journey. Sharing your experiences can help cultivate a sense of community and encourage positivity.

Engaging in activities that bring you joy and fulfillment can also enhance your mental well-being. Whether it's pursuing a hobby, volunteering, or spending time in nature, prioritize moments that make you feel happy and grounded. Remember, maintaining a positive mindset is an ongoing process, so be patient with yourself and celebrate small victories along the way.

Tips for Navigating Daily Challenges

Navigating daily challenges with endometriosis requires practical strategies to minimize disruptions. Start by establishing a routine that accommodates your symptoms. This may involve planning your activities around your energy levels, scheduling rest breaks, and incorporating light exercise to help manage pain. Communicate openly with your employer or school about your condition, allowing for flexibility when needed.

Additionally, prepare for challenging days by having a self-care kit on hand. Include items that help you cope with pain and fatigue, such as heat packs, pain relief medication, and calming herbal teas. Also, consider meal prepping to ensure you have nutritious meals ready to go, minimizing the stress of cooking on difficult days. Being proactive can help you feel more in control and reduce the impact of daily challenges.

Engaging in Self-Compassion and Self-Care

Self-compassion is essential for anyone managing a chronic condition like endometriosis. Acknowledge your struggles without judgment and treat yourself with kindness. This could mean allowing yourself to rest when needed or forgiving yourself for not meeting certain expectations. Practicing self-compassion can help alleviate feelings of frustration and guilt, fostering a healthier mindset.

Incorporating self-care practices into your routine is equally important. This can involve setting aside time for relaxation, whether through meditation, yoga, or simply taking a warm bath. Regularly engage in activities that nourish your body and mind, such as reading, art, or spending time in nature. Remember, self-care isn't selfish; it's a necessary part of managing your well-being.

Creating a Fulfilling Life with Endometriosis

Creating a fulfilling life while managing endometriosis involves prioritizing activities that bring joy and satisfaction. Start by identifying your passions and interests, whether they be artistic, athletic, or social. Set achievable goals that align with your interests and allow for flexibility based on your energy levels. Consider joining clubs or groups that share similar interests, as this can provide social support and enhance your sense of community.

Additionally, be open to exploring new opportunities that align with your values. This might mean pursuing a new career path, taking up a new hobby, or engaging in volunteer work. Embrace the idea that while endometriosis is part of your life, it doesn't define you; you have the power to create a fulfilling and meaningful life.

Resources for Ongoing Support and Education

Accessing resources for support and education is crucial in managing endometriosis effectively. Start by identifying reputable organizations and websites that offer information about the condition. Organizations such as the Endometriosis Foundation of America provide resources, research updates, and support networks for individuals affected by endometriosis.

Educational materials can empower you with knowledge about treatment options and self-management techniques.

In addition to online resources, consider joining local support groups or online forums where you can connect with others facing similar challenges. Sharing experiences and advice can provide comfort and practical insights. Attending workshops or seminars can also enhance your understanding of endometriosis and offer opportunities to learn from experts in the field.

Building Resilience and Coping Skills

Building resilience is vital for effectively managing the ups and downs of living with endometriosis. Start by developing coping skills that help you navigate difficult situations. This can include practicing mindfulness techniques, such as meditation or deep-breathing exercises, to help manage stress and anxiety. Keeping a journal to express your thoughts and feelings can also promote emotional resilience.

Moreover, focus on developing a support network that fosters resilience. Surround yourself with friends and family who understand your condition and can offer emotional support. Engaging in activities that promote personal growth and self-discovery can also enhance your resilience, allowing you to face challenges with a stronger mindset.

Importance of Long-Term Planning and Goal Setting

Long-term planning and goal setting are essential for managing endometriosis effectively. Start by identifying your personal health goals, whether they involve symptom management, career aspirations, or lifestyle changes. Break these goals into smaller, achievable steps to maintain motivation and focus. Regularly review your progress and adjust your goals as necessary to ensure they remain realistic and relevant.

Additionally, consider collaborating with your healthcare team to create a comprehensive long-term plan. Discuss potential treatments, lifestyle adjustments, and follow-up appointments that align with your goals. Establishing a clear plan helps provide structure and direction, making it easier to navigate the complexities of living with endometriosis.

Utilizing Technology for Health Management

Leveraging technology can significantly enhance your health management strategies for endometriosis. Start by exploring apps designed to track symptoms, medication, and menstrual cycles. These tools can provide insights into patterns and help you communicate effectively with your healthcare provider about your progress and experiences.

Social media can also be a valuable resource for finding support and information. Join online communities or follow educational accounts that focus on endometriosis. Engaging with others who share similar experiences can foster connection and provide access to resources, tips, and personal stories that may help you on your journey.

Celebrating Your Journey and Achievements

Celebrating your journey and achievements, no matter how small, is essential for maintaining motivation and positivity while managing endometriosis. Take time to reflect on the progress you have made, whether it's improvements in symptom management, personal growth, or milestones achieved. Recognize your resilience and strength in navigating the challenges associated with the condition.

Consider establishing a ritual for celebrating your successes, such as treating yourself to a special outing or indulging in a favorite activity. Sharing your accomplishments with supportive friends and family can amplify the joy of your achievements. Remember, celebrating your journey reinforces the notion that every step forward is significant, encouraging you to continue striving for a fulfilling life.

Staying Connected with the Endometriosis Community

Staying connected with the endometriosis community can provide valuable support and resources throughout your journey. Engage with local support groups, online forums, or social media platforms where individuals share their experiences and insights. Connecting with others who understand your challenges can foster a sense of belonging and reduce feelings of isolation.

Additionally, participate in awareness events, workshops, or advocacy efforts related to endometriosis. These activities not only provide opportunities to meet others but also contribute to raising awareness about the condition. Staying active within the community empowers you and can inspire change while providing ongoing education and support.

Common Concerns

1. Can endometriosis go away on its own?

Endometriosis is a complex condition that often does not resolve without intervention. Some individuals may experience temporary relief from symptoms, particularly during pregnancy or menopause, but this does not mean the endometriosis itself has disappeared. Regular monitoring and management are essential, as the condition can persist or worsen over time if left untreated.

To address endometriosis effectively, it's crucial to consult with a healthcare provider who can provide an accurate diagnosis and recommend a treatment plan tailored to your needs. Treatment options may include hormonal therapies, medications for pain relief, or surgical procedures to remove endometrial tissue. Staying proactive about your health can help manage symptoms and improve your quality of life.

2. What are the chances of getting pregnant with endometriosis?

The likelihood of conception with endometriosis varies depending on the severity of the condition. While endometriosis can cause fertility issues due to the formation of scar tissue or anatomical changes in the reproductive organs, many women with mild to moderate endometriosis can still conceive naturally. It's important to seek medical advice if you are trying to get pregnant, as a specialist can provide tailored treatment options.

Assisted reproductive technologies, such as in vitro fertilization (IVF), may also be recommended for those with more severe endometriosis or who have been unsuccessful in conceiving. Consulting a fertility specialist who understands the impacts of endometriosis can help optimize your chances of pregnancy.

3. Are there any natural remedies for endometriosis?

While natural remedies cannot cure endometriosis, they may help alleviate some symptoms. Options like heat therapy, including heating pads or hot baths, can provide temporary relief from pelvic pain. Herbal supplements, such as turmeric or ginger, have anti-inflammatory properties that may help reduce discomfort, but it's essential to consult a healthcare provider before starting any new treatment.

Incorporating mindfulness practices, such as yoga or meditation, can also be beneficial for managing stress and pain. A holistic approach that includes regular physical activity, relaxation techniques, and possibly acupuncture can complement medical treatments and enhance your overall well-being.

4. How does endometriosis affect my menstrual cycle?

Endometriosis can significantly impact the menstrual cycle, often leading to heavy, painful periods (dysmenorrhea). The presence of endometrial-like tissue outside the uterus responds to hormonal changes, causing inflammation and pain. You may also experience irregular cycles or spotting between periods, which can be distressing and impact your daily life.

Keeping a menstrual diary can help track your cycle, symptoms, and any patterns over time. Sharing this information with your healthcare provider can lead to more personalized treatment options to manage symptoms effectively, including pain management strategies and hormonal treatments.

5. What are the potential complications of untreated endometriosis?

Untreated endometriosis can lead to several complications, including chronic pain, infertility, and the development of ovarian cysts (endometriomas). The condition may also cause adhesions, which are bands of scar tissue that can bind organs together, leading to further pain and complications during surgery or childbirth.

It's crucial to monitor symptoms and seek treatment to minimize these risks. Early intervention can prevent complications and significantly improve your quality of life, helping you manage symptoms effectively and reduce the likelihood of infertility.

6. How can I find a specialist for endometriosis?

Finding a specialist for endometriosis begins with your primary care physician or gynecologist, who can provide referrals to professionals experienced in treating this condition. Look for providers who have expertise in endometriosis management, such as reproductive endocrinologists, gynecologic surgeons, or pain specialists. Researching their credentials, experience, and patient reviews can also help in your selection.

Consider seeking a multidisciplinary team approach, which may include physical therapists, nutritionists, and mental health professionals to address the various aspects of endometriosis. Patient advocacy groups and online communities can also provide recommendations and support in your search for specialized care.

7. What lifestyle changes can improve my symptoms?

Implementing lifestyle changes can help manage endometriosis symptoms effectively. Regular exercise promotes overall health and can reduce inflammation and stress, which may alleviate pain. Focus on a balanced diet rich in fruits, vegetables, whole grains, and lean proteins to support your immune system and reduce inflammation.

Additionally, establishing a regular sleep routine and incorporating stress management techniques, such as mindfulness or yoga, can contribute to improved symptom control. Keeping a symptom diary to track triggers can also help you identify specific lifestyle factors that may worsen your condition, allowing you to make more informed adjustments.

8. How do I cope with the emotional impact of endometriosis?

Coping with the emotional toll of endometriosis can be challenging, but support is available. Connecting with support groups, either in person or online, allows you to share experiences and learn from others facing similar struggles. This sense of community can provide validation and encouragement during difficult times.

Additionally, consider speaking with a mental health professional who specializes in chronic illness or reproductive health. Therapy can help you develop coping strategies for managing anxiety, depression, or feelings of isolation related to endometriosis. Open communication with friends and family about your experiences can also foster understanding and support.

9. Are there any dietary recommendations for endometriosis?

Dietary changes may help alleviate endometriosis symptoms and improve overall health. Focus on an anti-inflammatory diet, which includes plenty of fruits, vegetables, whole grains, healthy fats, and lean proteins. Omega-3 fatty acids found in fatty fish, walnuts, and flaxseeds can be particularly beneficial in reducing inflammation.

Avoiding processed foods, excessive sugar, and trans fats can also support better health. Keeping a food diary can help you identify any foods that may trigger your symptoms, allowing you to make informed dietary choices tailored to your needs. Consulting a nutritionist familiar with endometriosis can provide personalized guidance.

10. How can I manage endometriosis during pregnancy?

Managing endometriosis during pregnancy requires careful planning and collaboration with your healthcare provider. While many women with endometriosis can have healthy pregnancies, some may experience increased pain or complications. It's essential to communicate openly about your history and any symptoms you may have during pregnancy.

Pain management strategies may include safe medications approved by your healthcare provider. Engaging in light exercise, practicing relaxation techniques, and maintaining a nutritious diet can also help manage symptoms. Regular prenatal check-ups are vital for monitoring both your health and the health of your baby.

11. What surgical treatment options are available for endometriosis?

Surgical treatment for endometriosis aims to remove as much endometrial tissue as possible while preserving reproductive function. Laparoscopy is a common minimally invasive procedure that allows the surgeon to visualize and remove endometriosis lesions. In more severe cases, a laparotomy may be required for extensive tissue removal.

If fertility is a concern, your surgeon may also recommend procedures that enhance your chances of conception. Discussing your options with a specialist can help determine the best course of action based on your individual circumstances and goals for treatment.

12. How can I monitor my endometriosis symptoms effectively?

Monitoring your endometriosis symptoms involves keeping a detailed diary to track menstrual cycles, pain levels, and other symptoms. This information can help you and your healthcare provider identify patterns and triggers, leading to more effective management strategies. Note any changes in your symptoms, lifestyle factors, and treatments to better understand what works for you.

Utilizing apps designed for tracking menstrual health can simplify this process. Regular follow-up appointments with your healthcare provider to discuss your diary findings can facilitate informed decisions about treatment options, lifestyle changes, and symptom management techniques.

13. What are the latest advancements in endometriosis research?

Recent advancements in endometriosis research focus on improving diagnostic techniques and treatment options. Non-invasive imaging methods, such as MRI, are being explored to enhance early detection of endometriosis. Genetic and molecular research aims to understand the underlying causes of the condition better and develop targeted therapies.

Clinical trials are ongoing to evaluate new medical treatments, including hormone therapies and immunotherapies, which may offer improved symptom relief. Staying informed about these advancements through reputable medical sources can empower you to discuss new options with your healthcare provider, ensuring that you have access to the latest treatment strategies.

Detailed FAQs

How Endometriosis Develops

Endometriosis occurs when tissue similar to the lining of the uterus grows outside it, commonly on the ovaries, fallopian tubes, and pelvic lining. This tissue responds to hormonal changes during the menstrual cycle, leading to inflammation, pain, and scar tissue formation. Factors like retrograde menstruation, where menstrual blood flows backward through the fallopian tubes, and immune system disorders are believed to contribute to the development of this condition.

To understand the development process, consider the role of hormones, particularly estrogen. During menstruation, the tissue outside the uterus thickens and sheds, similar to the uterine lining. However, unlike the lining, this tissue has no way to exit the body, causing inflammation and pain. Recognizing the hormonal aspect is key to grasping how endometriosis progresses and affects the body.

Common Symptoms to Watch For

Women with endometriosis often experience a range of symptoms, the most common being pelvic pain, which may occur during menstruation, intercourse, or bowel movements. Other symptoms can include heavy menstrual bleeding, fatigue, and gastrointestinal issues such as diarrhea or constipation. It's crucial to track these symptoms as they can help in understanding the severity and impact on daily life.

Keeping a symptom diary can be a practical tool for recognizing patterns. Note when symptoms occur, their intensity, and any potential triggers. This information can be invaluable during medical consultations, allowing healthcare providers to better assess the situation and develop effective management strategies.

Different Stages of Endometriosis

Endometriosis is classified into four stages: minimal, mild, moderate, and severe, based on the extent of the tissue growth and the presence of adhesions. Stage I (minimal) has small implants, while Stage IV (severe) presents with deep, large lesions and significant adhesions. Understanding these stages helps women identify their condition's severity and inform treatment decisions.

Women can discuss these stages with their healthcare provider during diagnosis. This conversation should focus on the specific characteristics of their endometriosis, as well as possible treatment options based on the stage. Knowing the stage can aid in creating personalized management plans.

Risk Factors Associated with the Condition

Certain risk factors may increase the likelihood of developing endometriosis, including family history, early menstruation, short menstrual cycles, and prolonged estrogen exposure. Additionally, lifestyle factors like high body weight and low physical activity may also play a role. Recognizing these risk factors can empower women to take proactive steps in managing their reproductive health.

To mitigate these risks, women should consider lifestyle changes, such as maintaining a healthy weight through a balanced diet and regular exercise. Regular check-ups with healthcare providers can also help monitor reproductive health, especially for those with a family history of endometriosis.

How Endometriosis Is Diagnosed

Diagnosing endometriosis typically involves a combination of pelvic exams, imaging tests like ultrasounds, and laparoscopy, a minimally invasive surgical procedure. During laparoscopy, a surgeon can view the pelvic organs and, if necessary, take biopsies for further examination. It's important for women to advocate for themselves if they suspect endometriosis, as it can sometimes be overlooked.

For those experiencing persistent symptoms, seeking a second opinion can be beneficial. Discussing symptoms openly with a healthcare provider and expressing concerns about endometriosis can lead to appropriate diagnostic measures, ensuring a comprehensive evaluation.

Importance of Early Detection

Early detection of endometriosis is crucial for effective management and improving quality of life. Women who recognize symptoms early are more likely to receive timely treatment, which can help alleviate pain and address fertility concerns. Additionally, early intervention can prevent the progression of the disease and the development of severe symptoms.

Women should prioritize regular gynecological check-ups and maintain open communication with their healthcare providers about any changes in their reproductive health. Staying informed and proactive can significantly enhance outcomes related to endometriosis management.

Impact on Daily Life

Endometriosis can profoundly affect daily life, influencing physical activities, work performance, and emotional well-being. Women may experience debilitating pain, fatigue, and mental health challenges, leading to missed work or social engagements. Understanding this impact is essential for developing effective coping strategies and seeking support.

To navigate these challenges, women are encouraged to build a support network, including friends, family, and healthcare professionals. Self-care practices, such as mindfulness, stress management, and regular exercise, can also help improve overall well-being and reduce the emotional toll of the condition.

Myths and Misconceptions

There are many myths surrounding endometriosis, including misconceptions that it only affects women who are infertile or that it always presents with severe pain. Such misconceptions can lead to stigma and misunderstandings, preventing women from seeking the help they need. Education and awareness are vital to dispelling these myths.

To combat misinformation, women should seek reliable sources of information, such as healthcare providers or reputable organizations dedicated to reproductive health. Engaging in discussions about endometriosis can help raise awareness and foster a more supportive environment for those affected.

Connection between Endometriosis and Other Health Issues

Endometriosis is often linked to other health issues, such as infertility, ovarian cysts, and autoimmune disorders. Understanding these connections can help women recognize the broader implications of their condition and encourage comprehensive healthcare. It's important for women to discuss these potential associations with their healthcare providers.

Maintaining a holistic view of health can aid in addressing related concerns. Women may benefit from integrative approaches that consider both endometriosis and any associated health issues, ensuring a more thorough management plan that addresses overall well-being.

Current Statistics and Prevalence

Endometriosis affects an estimated 1 in 10 women of reproductive age, highlighting its significance as a widespread condition. Awareness of these statistics can encourage women to seek help and validate their experiences, knowing they are not alone. Understanding the prevalence can also support advocacy efforts for better research and treatment options.

Women can use these statistics to raise awareness in their communities and advocate for greater resources and research funding. Sharing personal stories and statistics can help break the silence surrounding endometriosis and promote a more supportive environment for those affected.

Resources for Further Learning

Numerous resources are available for women seeking to learn more about endometriosis. Reputable organizations, books, and online forums can provide valuable information and support. These resources can empower women to understand their condition better and connect with others facing similar challenges.

Exploring local support groups or online communities can also foster a sense of belonging and provide opportunities for sharing experiences. Engaging with these resources can enhance knowledge and offer practical advice for managing endometriosis.

Importance of Patient Advocacy

Patient advocacy is crucial for women with endometriosis to ensure they receive the appropriate care and support. Being informed about their rights and options enables women to actively participate in their healthcare decisions. Advocacy can lead to better treatment outcomes and increased awareness about the condition.

Women can become advocates by educating themselves and others about endometriosis, sharing their experiences, and participating in awareness campaigns. Collaborating with healthcare professionals and organizations can help amplify their voices and push for necessary changes in endometriosis research and treatment.

Conclusion

In conclusion, understanding and managing endometriosis is crucial for improving the quality of life for those affected. By learning about the condition, recognizing symptoms, and seeking appropriate support, women can take proactive steps towards effective management. From pain relief strategies to fertility support and surgical options, this resource serves as a comprehensive guide. Emphasizing the importance of advocacy, emotional support, and lifestyle modifications, we hope to empower women to navigate their journey with endometriosis confidently. Remember, you are not alone—connect with others, seek help, and take charge of your health.